The characters and events in this book are Non-fiction.

This book is not intended as a substitue for the medical advice of physicians.

The reader should regularly consult a physician in matters relating to

his/her health and particularly with respect to any symptoms that may require

diagnosis or medical attention.

Library of Congress Cataloging-in-Publication Data

Lee, V Tracy.

Exercising The Brain Down Memory Lane "A Guideline To Remember" / Tracy V Lee. —1st ed.

p. cm.

ISBN-13: 978-1729729915

1.Biography —Non-fiction.

Printed in the United States of America

Cover design by Sahara Coleman

"This book is dedicated to my late father Lucien Lee with love."

Who was dealing with dementia and had been for about five years before he passed away in early 2018.

Through it all, my daughter and I have been there with him as his caregivers. He was the one who inspired me to take a chance and put this book together for others who might be going through the same thing or need something to do.

He was a Veteran, Husband, Father, and Grandfather. He was all around a hilarious man, who is genuinely missed dearly.

Rest in Peace Father.

-Your Affectionate Daughter

Tracy V. Lee

A Book not just for the "Common Illness" but for all of those who want to sustain, maintain and improve your mind. To find the strength to be the best you can be.

The Secret to an extraordinary life is "Staying Busy."

*Like I said before, my Dad had dementia. The doctor told him to stay busy. It will help slow down the rapid progress of the illness. However, my Dad had other plans. All he wanted to do was sleep through the day and walk around all night (Sundowning).

Here are a few ways to "Staying Busy":

- **Exercise**- such as; going for a walk, planting a garden, cleaning/organizing, dancing and jogging/running.
- **Games**- such as; crossword puzzles, playing a sport, video games, card games, family games
- **Reading, Writing, Drawing**
- **Join a Day Center**- It offers benefits to all in need of physical, mental, and emotional care. It provides services such as; counseling, health services, personal nutrition care, activities, behavior management, therapy, and special needs.

"Anything That Challenges Your Mind"

“I Am Never Alone. As Long As I Keep God First”

# Table of Contents

*Blank Pages will be a space left open for your creativity*

# Appointment Reminder Fill-In

| Date: | Date: | Date: |
| Time: | Time: | Time: |

| Date: | Date: | Date: |
| Time: | Time: | Time: |

| Date: | Date: | Date: |
| Time: | Time: | Time: |

| Date: | Date: | Date: |
| Time: | Time: | Time: |

| Date: | Date: | Date: |
| Time: | Time: | Time: |

| Date: | Date: | Date: |
| Time: | Time: | Time: |

| Date: | Date: | Date: |
| Time: | Time: | Time: |

# Journal Notes
(Your Journal Entries Below)

# <u>Crossword Puzzle</u>

(Fill- in puzzle across/up/down by using the sentences below that explain each word. Check your answer below)

<u>Across</u>

1. Refusing to be persuaded or to change one's mind
2. Undergo great mental anguish through worrying about something
3. Give Knowledge or understanding of something
4. Not having or showing the necessary skills to do something successfully
5. To perceive or point out a difference

<u>Down</u>

6. Leave out or exclude someone/something, either intentionally or forgetfully
7. Protection of or authority over someone or something; guardianship
8. Become aware or conscious of something/someone; come to realize or understand
9. To participate or become involved in

"Check bottom of next page for answers"

| | | | |
|---|---|---|---|
| 1. | Adamant | 6. | Omit |
| 2. | Agonize | 7. | Tutelage |
| 3. | Familiarize | 8. | Perceive |
| 4. | Incompetent | 9. | Engage |
| 5. | Distinguish | | |

# Coloring Page

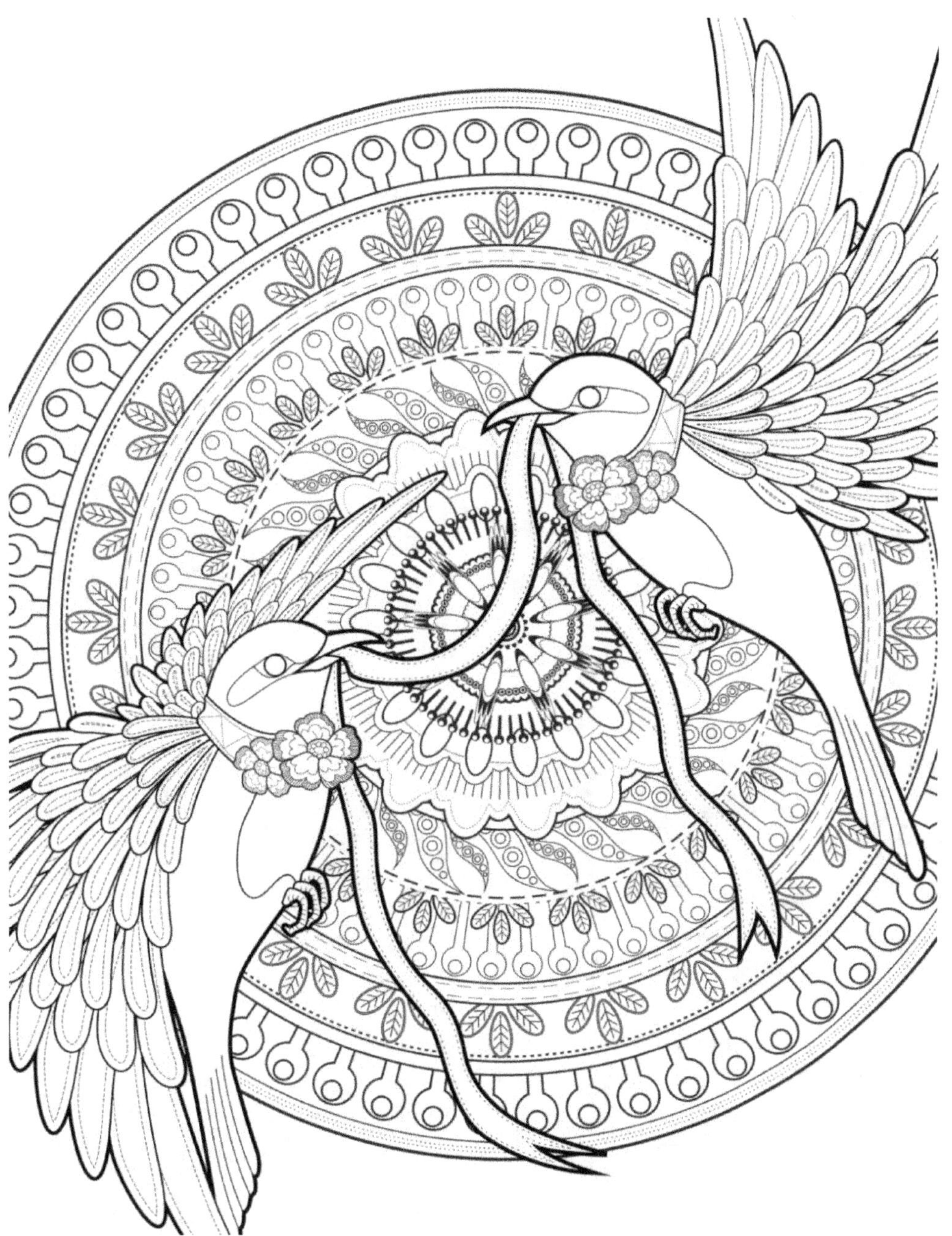

"Birds of a Feather That Flock Together"

# List Of Pros and Cons

# Appointment Reminder Fill-In

| Date: | Date: | Date: |
|---|---|---|
| Time: | Time: | Time: |

| Date: | Date: | Date: |
|---|---|---|
| Time: | Time: | Time: |

| Date: | Date: | Date: |
|---|---|---|
| Time: | Time: | Time: |

| Date: | Date: | Date: |
|---|---|---|
| Time: | Time: | Time: |

| Date: | Date: | Date: |
|---|---|---|
| Time: | Time: | Time: |

| Date: | Date: | Date: |
|---|---|---|
| Time: | Time: | Time: |

| Date: | Date: | Date: |
|---|---|---|
| Time: | Time: | Time: |

| Date: | Date: | Date: |
|---|---|---|
| Time: | Time: | Time: |

# Journal Notes
### (Your Journal Entries Below)

# <u>Word Search</u>

```
B R A I N W R E C K G K N M N N U I O J K L P
E R E T E W R G L O V E S M A R T S E E K R L
A R G U E F I G H T F O R G E T S U N D O W N
E R S S A D L O S T F I N D F O U N D G O N E
M E M O R Y B R A V E S A M E F O R E V E R
L O N G T E R M S T R O K E B R E A T H I N G
H E A R T A C H E P S Y C H O L O G Y O L O G
G E T O U T R E T R I E V E L O O S E N E V E R
S A Y N E V E R A B I L I T Y T O W O N D E R I
```

- Someone who has advanced in years
- Where information is encoded, stored and retrieved
- To bring awareness of something/someone to one's mind
- Possession of the means or skill to do something
- To bring something back into one's mind
- Covering the hands worn for protection against cold or dirt
- To cause destruction of something by sinking or breaking up
- No longer present; departed
- Attempt or desire to find something or someone
- A muscular organ which pumps blood through the blood vessels of the circulatory system

"Check bottom of next page for answers"

| | |
|---|---|
| • Brain | • Gloves |
| • Long Term | • Wreck |
| • Ability | • Gone |
| • Retrieve | • Seek |
| • Psychology | • Heart |

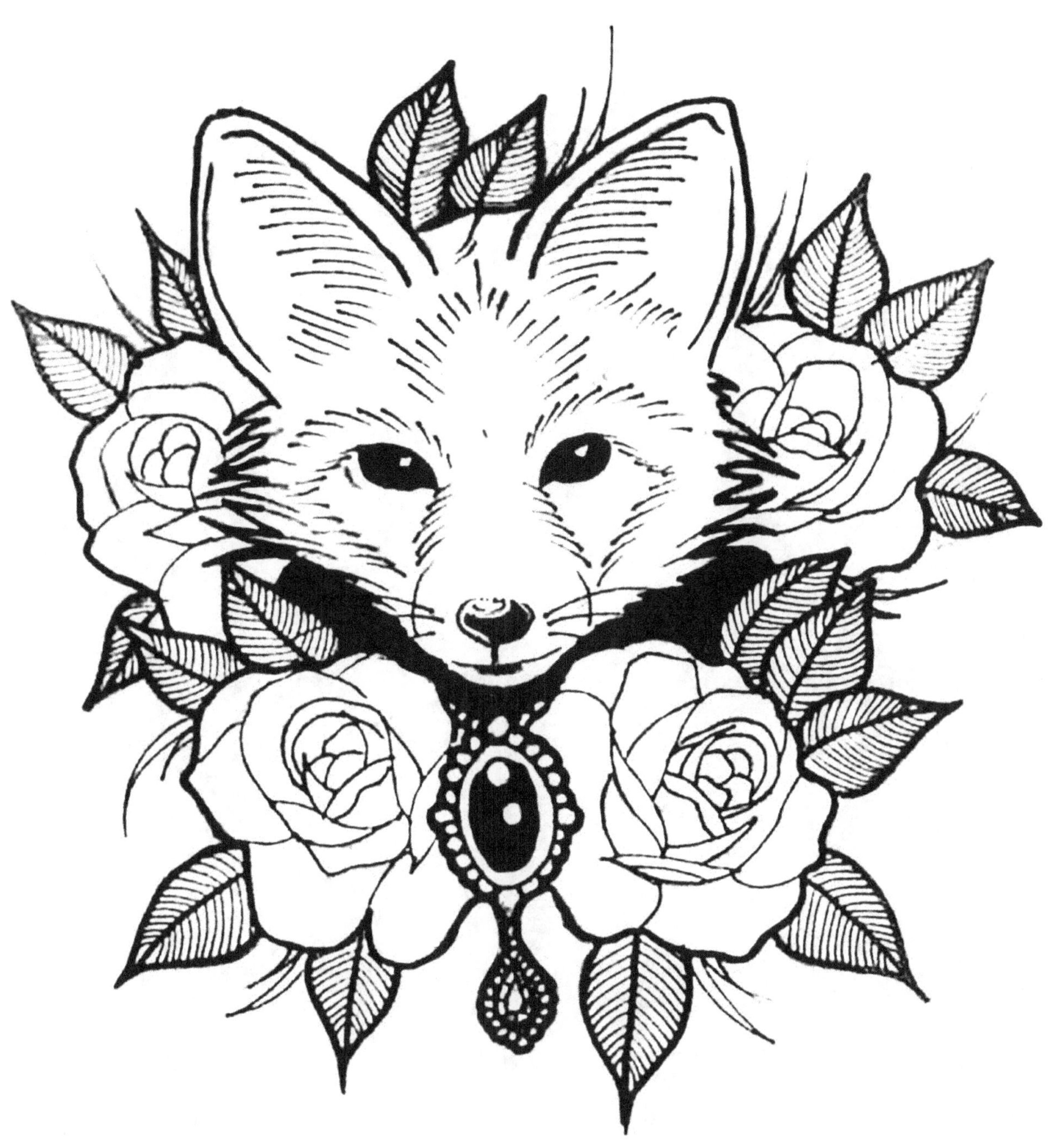

"Sly Fox Bejeweled"

<u>**List Of Pros and Cons**</u>

# <u>Coloring Page</u>

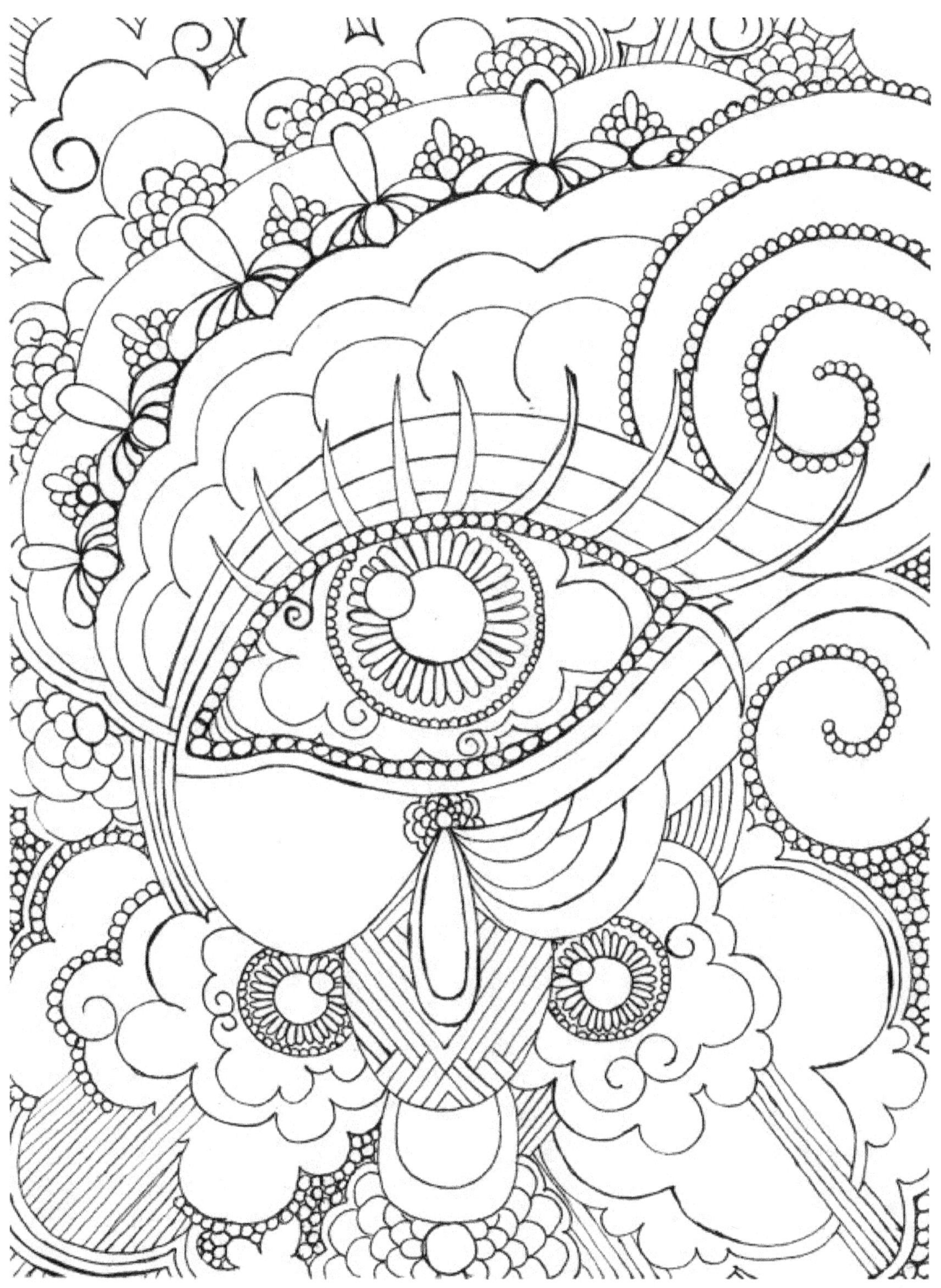

"In the eye of the beholder"

# <u>Counting Numbers</u>

(Count from 1 to 100 then backwards from 100 to 1)

## Counting Chart: Numbers 1 to 100

| 1<br>one | 2<br>two | 3<br>three | 4<br>four | 5<br>five | 6<br>six | 7<br>seven | 8<br>eight | 9<br>nine | 10<br>ten |
|---|---|---|---|---|---|---|---|---|---|
| 11<br>eleven | 12<br>twelve | 13<br>thirteen | 14<br>fourteen | 15<br>fifteen | 16<br>sixteen | 17<br>seventeen | 18<br>eighteen | 19<br>nineteen | 20<br>twenty |
| 21<br>twenty-one | 22<br>twenty-two | 23<br>twenty-three | 24<br>twenty-four | 25<br>twenty-five | 26<br>twenty-six | 27<br>twenty-seven | 28<br>twenty-eight | 29<br>twenty-nine | 30<br>thirty |
| 31<br>thirty-one | 32<br>thirty-two | 33<br>thirty-three | 34<br>thirty-four | 35<br>thirty-five | 36<br>thirty-six | 37<br>thirty-seven | 38<br>thirty-eight | 39<br>thirty-nine | 40<br>forty |
| 41<br>forty-one | 42<br>forty-two | 43<br>forty-three | 44<br>forty-four | 45<br>forty-five | 46<br>forty-six | 47<br>forty-seven | 48<br>forty-eight | 49<br>forty-nine | 50<br>fifty |
| 51<br>fifty-one | 52<br>fifty-two | 53<br>fifty-three | 54<br>fifty-four | 55<br>fifty-five | 56<br>fifty-six | 57<br>fifty-seven | 58<br>fifty-eight | 59<br>fifty-nine | 60<br>sixty |
| 61<br>sixty-one | 62<br>sixty-two | 63<br>sixty-three | 64<br>sixty-four | 65<br>sixty-five | 66<br>sixty-six | 67<br>sixty-seven | 68<br>sixty-eight | 69<br>sixty-nine | 70<br>seventy |
| 71<br>seventy-one | 72<br>seventy-two | 73<br>seventy-three | 74<br>seventy-four | 75<br>seventy-five | 76<br>seventy-six | 77<br>seventy-seven | 78<br>seventy-eight | 79<br>seventy-nine | 80<br>eighty |
| 81<br>eighty-one | 82<br>eighty-two | 83<br>eighty-three | 84<br>eighty-four | 85<br>eighty-five | 86<br>eighty-six | 87<br>eighty-seven | 88<br>eighty-eight | 89<br>eighty-nine | 90<br>ninety |
| 91<br>ninety-one | 92<br>ninety-two | 93<br>ninety-three | 94<br>ninety-four | 95<br>ninety-five | 96<br>ninety-six | 97<br>ninety-seven | 98<br>ninety-eight | 99<br>ninety-nine | 100<br>one hundred |

# <u>Brain Teasers</u>

(Which one doesn't belong? Fill- in answer in blank. When finished, check bottom of next page for answers)

a)

- ❖ Sophisticated
- ❖ High-Class
- ❖ Vulgar
- ❖ Upscale

________________________

b)

- ❖ Rolls-Royce
- ❖ Jaguar
- ❖ Bentley
- ❖ Genesis

________________________

c)

- ❖ Archery
- ❖ Polo Ralph Lauren
- ❖ Hockey
- ❖ Golf

________________________

d)

- ❖ Apple
- ❖ Banana
- ❖ Orange
- ❖ Pear

________________________

a) Vulgar
b) Jaguar( Can be a car or animal
c) Polo Ralph Lauren (Polo is a sport. Ralph Lauren is the clothing brand)
d) Orange(Fruit or Color)

# <u>Unscramble</u>

(Unscramble the sentences by placing the words in correct order. When finished, check bottom of next page for answers.)

A)

- o  "Garden to tend to time the"

B)

- o  "All the complete of words you can?"

C)

- o  "Count can you on me"

D)

- o  "The same doing appear to be people with higher incomes."

|     |                                              |
| --- | -------------------------------------------- |
| A)  | Time to tend to the garden.                  |
| B)  | Can you complete all of the words?           |
| C)  | You can count on me                          |
| D)  | People with higher incomes appear to be doing the same |

# Workshop Exercise Part 1
### (Daily Reminder)

Date:

Time:

Name:

Address:

Favorite Food:

Age:

Gender:

# <u>Workshop Exercise Part 1</u>
(Daily Reminder)

Date:

Time:

Mother's Name:

Father's Name:

Favorite Movie:

What Did You Have For Breakfast, Lunch, and Dinner? :

What Country, State, City, and Town Do You Live In? :

# Workshop Exercise Part 2
(Write down your favorite thing's)

# Workshop Exercise Part 2

(Write down your favorite thing's)

# <u>Workshop Exercise Part 3</u>

(Goals Workshop-Develop your goals)
"Make a list of goals, next to each one write down the
time in which you can commit to accomplishing them"

|  |  |
| --- | --- |
|  |  |
|  |  |
|  |  |
|  |  |
|  |  |
|  |  |
|  |  |
|  |  |
|  |  |
|  |  |
|  |  |
|  |  |
|  |  |
|  |  |
|  |  |
|  |  |
|  |  |
|  |  |
|  |  |
|  |  |
|  |  |
|  |  |

# <u>Workshop Exercise Part 3</u>

(Goals Workshop-Develop your goals)

"Make a list of goals, next to each one write down the
time in which you can commit to accomplishing them"

|  |  |
| --- | --- |
|  |  |
|  |  |
|  |  |
|  |  |
|  |  |
|  |  |
|  |  |
|  |  |
|  |  |
|  |  |
|  |  |
|  |  |
|  |  |
|  |  |
|  |  |
|  |  |
|  |  |
|  |  |
|  |  |
|  |  |
|  |  |
|  |  |

# Workshop Exercise Part 4

(Behavior Problems)
"Write down when you've had a bad day and why?"

# <u>Workshop Exercise Part 4</u>

(Behavior Problems)

"Write down when you've had a bad day and why?"

# <u>Workshop Exercise Part 5</u>

(Challenge your memory)

"Write a short story. It could be about yourself, a friend, or family."

# Workshop Exercise Part 5

(Challenge your memory)
"Write a short story. It could be about yourself, a friend, or family."

# <u>Workshop Exercise Part 6</u>

(The Good vs. The Bad)

- Step 1: Make a list of all of the things that make you feel "good" about yourself

_______________________________________________________

_______________________________________________________

_______________________________________________________

_______________________________________________________

_______________________________________________________

_______________________________________________________

- Step 2: Make a list of all of the things that make you feel "bad" about yourself

_______________________________________________________

_______________________________________________________

_______________________________________________________

_______________________________________________________

_______________________________________________________

_______________________________________________________

"When you've completed your list, show it to your caregiver, guardian or doctor if you like."

# <u>Workshop Exercise Part 6</u>

(The Good vs The Bad)

- Step 1: Make a list of all of the things that make you feel "good" about yourself

________________________________________________________

________________________________________________________

________________________________________________________

________________________________________________________

________________________________________________________

- Step 2: Make a list of all of the things that make you feel "bad" about yourself

________________________________________________________

________________________________________________________

________________________________________________________

________________________________________________________

________________________________________________________

"When you've completed your list, show it to your caregiver, guardian or doctor if you like."

# <u>Workshop Exercise Part 7</u>

(Keeping Busy)

"Make a list of all the activities you can do to stay busy and keep you happy."

# <u>Workshop Exercise Part 7</u>

(Keeping Busy)

"Make a list of all the activities you can do to stay busy and keep you happy."

# <u>Workshop Exercise Part 8</u>

(Health)
"Make a workout schedule and what you eat/drink on that day as well."

## Weekly Schedule

| Sun | Mon | Tue | Wed | Thu | Fri | Sat |
|-----|-----|-----|-----|-----|-----|-----|
|     |     |     |     |     |     |     |
|     |     |     |     |     |     |     |
|     |     |     |     |     |     |     |
|     |     |     |     |     |     |     |
|     |     |     |     |     |     |     |

# <u>Workshop Exercise Part 8</u>

(Health)

"Make a workout schedule and what you eat/drink on that day as well."

## Weekly Schedule

| Sun | Mon | Tue | Wed | Thu | Fri | Sat |
|-----|-----|-----|-----|-----|-----|-----|
|     |     |     |     |     |     |     |
|     |     |     |     |     |     |     |
|     |     |     |     |     |     |     |
|     |     |     |     |     |     |     |
|     |     |     |     |     |     |     |
|     |     |     |     |     |     |     |